WHAT YOUR GYNECOLOGIST NEVER TOLD YOU...
AND YOUR MOTHER DIDN'T KNOW

*Everything You Need To Know Before
Your Next Gynecologic Visit*

Tara A. Solomon, M.D.

AuthorHouse™
1663 Liberty Drive, Suite 200
Bloomington, IN 47403
www.authorhouse.com
Phone: 1-800-839-8640

This book should not replace medical advice from a physician. The
author is not responsible for any liability that occurs as a consequence
of the use or application of any of the contents of this book.

First published by AuthorHouse 10/7/2008

ISBN: 978-1-4389-1479-4 (sc)
ISBN: 978-1-4389-1480-0 (hc)

Library of Congress Control Number: 2008908138

Printed in the United States of America
Bloomington, Indiana

This book is printed on acid-free paper.

Dedication

To my mother, the late Sharyn Solomon, whose compassion, devotion, and love inspired me to write this book.

I wish you were here.

Table of Contents

Introduction

Twelve years of practicing obstetrics and gynecology and more than 100,000 patients later, I have discovered that there is not enough time during a patient encounter to thoroughly discuss women's health issues. Decreasing reimbursement rates from insurance companies and increasing overhead costs have forced many physicians to limit the amount of time spent face-to-face with patients. Women are often left "doctor-hopping" until they can find a solution to their health problem.

As I was writing **What Your Gynecologist Never Told You ... And Your Mother Didn't Know,** I was astounded by the technological and pharmaceutical advances over the last decade that are helping women lead healthier, more productive lives.

In this book, I will share with you a wealth of information concerning women's health issues that have surfaced over and over again in my practice. With this knowledge base, you can take control of your health, focus on health care problems that may be interfering with your quality of life, and learn ways to prevent diseases that strike many women in their golden years.

Read this book before you make your next gynecological appointment. You will be pleasantly surprised at how much more you will benefit from your next visit. Here's to a happy and healthy life!

Tara A. Solomon, MD, FACOG

Chapter 1

What to Expect From a Routine Annual Checkup

The dreaded annual gyn exam—this is what most of my patients think when they get their appointment reminder cards in the mail. By the time their exam is done, they say to me, "That wasn't so bad!" Your annual gynecologic exam should be a pleasant experience. Just make sure that you are well prepared to ask pertinent questions and show your physician anything that you feel is out of the ordinary.

When a woman makes an appointment for an annual checkup or "well-woman exam," as the physician's office codes the visit, she should be sure that a pertinent history is taken. A certain number of items should be performed in a basic physical examination, blood work should be taken, and referrals should be given for pertinent radiological testing and specialty consultations.

I always begin an annual checkup face-to-face, with my patient seated in my office. I find that this tends to break the ice. Do not let a physician whom you have never met interview you for the first time with your legs up in stirrups. This is both unprofessional and discourteous. The first thing that we will discuss is the reason for the patient's visit. Is she here for an annual checkup without any physical or emotional complaints or does she have a problem with her menstrual cycles or menopausal hot flashes? Make sure that you have written down your complaints and questions before reaching the doctor's office, so that you will not forget the information under the pressure of an office visit.

I will then ask pertinent information about her medical history, such as diabetes, high blood pressure, asthma, thyroid disease, any allergies pertaining to certain food and medications, and medications that she may be taking, as well as over-the-counter vitamins, herbs, and other supplements. Herbs and supplements have become such a routine in my patients' diets that they often forget to disclose this information. Herbal remedies can have severe interactions with pharmaceuticals, so please let your doctor know about them.

Next, I proceed with a discussion about a patient's surgical history, obstetrical history, and social history, which includes tobacco use, alcohol use, and illegal drug use. I will also ask about a patient's marital status and present sexual activity. Lastly but very importantly, we will end the conversation with a discussion about the patient's family history. This includes the family history of "first-degree" relatives, such as mother, father, sisters, and brothers, and also a family history of extended family members. My patients are often awestruck when they realize that they can genetically inherit a disease such as breast cancer from their father's side of the family! I cannot emphasize enough how important it is to know one's family history of stroke, heart attack, pulmonary embolus (blood clot in the lung), and deep venous thrombosis before asking your gynecologist for birth control or hormone replacement therapy for the first time. It could save your life!

The next part of the visit includes the physical examination. Make sure that you have emptied your bladder before undressing for your exam. This will make your exam much more comfortable. Ask the doctor if he or she needs a urine sample before you use the bathroom. If your gynecologist happens to be male, please ensure that there is a chaperone in the room with you. The law requires this, so do not feel intimidated to ask for a nurse or medical assistant if he walks into the room alone. You may also ask for a chaperone if your gynecologist is a woman. Make sure that you are completely covered from your neck down to your knees before your exam begins.

A routine exam begins with an examination of the head, eyes, ears, nose, and throat. Next, a thorough examination of the neck, including the thyroid gland and lymph nodes, is performed. I will often find a nodule on the thyroid gland or a lymph node in the neck that may lead to a further work-up. I continue the examination with a thorough breast examination, first with my patient sitting up and then with her lying down. Make sure to point out any areas of concern to your gynecologist, including nipple discharge, any painful areas or lumps, and any discolorations.

The examination continues with a heart and lung exam and then proceeds to an abdominal exam. I complete the exam with a pelvic examination, Pap smear, and recto-vaginal exam. My patients are often caught off guard by a rectal exam; however, this is an essential part of every gynecological exam. A gynecologist can find an unsuspected colorectal cancer; I have examined a woman just forty-two years old with anal cancer. The rectal exam can also uncover a small amount of blood in the stool (known as a Hemoccult® test). This microscopic quantity of blood in the stool may signal possible bowel disease such as Crohn's disease or ulcerative colitis.

Pap smears are performed yearly on sexually active women from the time of first sexual activity or age twenty-one until the age of sixty-five years. Since the causative agent of cervical cancer is human papillomavirus (HPV), a sexually transmitted disease, the American College of Obstetrics and Gynecology recently made the recommendation to stop annual Pap smears at the age of sixty-five years unless a woman is sexually active with a new partner or has a history of cervical cancer. Do not fall for the false assumption that menopause makes you immune to sexually transmitted diseases (STDs). I have seen a wide array of STDs in my female patients over fifty, from herpes to hepatitis C. Sexually active, non-monogamous women should be tested for gonorrhea, chlamydia, HIV, and herpes on an annual basis.

Once the physical examination has been completed, your gynecologist should counsel you on either birth control if you are in your reproductive years or hormone replacement therapy and/or calcium supplementation if you are menopausal. You may be asked to return for a follow-up visit to discuss your options if time does not permit.

Lastly, you should be given a prescription for an annual mammogram between the ages of thirty-five and forty for a screening mammogram, and then once a year when you reach the age of forty. Bone density studies should begin at the time of menopause and be repeated every two years afterward. Women begin to lose bone at the age of thirty, but a more rapid decline in bone loss occurs when they reach menopause. Screening colonoscopies should begin at the age of fifty, and if normal, be repeated every ten years.

If time permits and your physician performs blood drawing in the office, you should check the following blood work on an annual basis: thyroid function testing, fasting glucose, and lipid profile, including triglycerides, complete blood count (which checks your red blood cell count), metabolic panel (which checks your liver function and kidney function), and more recently added, a c-reactive protein which could point out an increased risk for heart disease, even at a young age. This concludes your annual examination. Most of the above history and physical takes place in a mere fifteen minutes in a typical gynecologist's office! This is why it is so important to come into your visit prepared to ask questions and point out physical ailments that would otherwise be overlooked during your brief encounter with the doctor.

Chapter 2

Birth Control: Myths vs. Realities

A patient recently came to me for a routine gynecologic exam. She was a non-smoking thirty-six-year-old mother of three who had been doing very well on birth control pills for the past ten years. She requested information about a bilateral tubal ligation (commonly known as "tying her tubes"). When I asked her what was wrong with her present method of contraception, she told me that she was too old to be taking the pill and that she feared that the pills may harm her body or give her cancer after so many years of use.

This scenario has become all too common in gynecologists' offices today. A majority of women believe that oral contraception serves only one purpose: pregnancy prevention. Little has been done to promote the multitude of preventive health care benefits of oral contraceptives, patches, and the birth control ring to patients and to dispel the many myths about birth control that have been handed down from generation to generation.

Let me share with you some of the most common misconceptions about birth control that I have heard over the years and my attempts to dispel them.

MYTH: Birth control pills cause cancer.

REALITY: Since the advent of low-dose oral contraceptive pills (OCPs) in the 1970s (as opposed to the higher dosage of estrogen contained in OCPs of prior years), no causal relationship has been proven between OCPs and ovarian or uterine cancer. In fact, birth control use of greater than ten years' duration has been associated with an 80 percent reduction in the risk of ovarian cancer and a 50 percent reduction in the risk of uterine cancer. That's right, birth control can *protect* you from cancer. Furthermore, the Collaborative Group on Epidemiological Studies of Ovarian Cancer published their study on the relationship between oral contraceptives and ovarian cancer in 2008 and found that oral contraceptives provide protection against ovarian cancer for up to thirty years or more after women stop taking them. Their findings show that birth control pills have prevented approximately 200,000 ovarian cancers and 100,000 deaths from the disease. Although most studies have not shown a correlation between birth control and breast cancer, a few have shown a slight increase in breast cancer in women with first-degree relatives with breast cancer.

A small but significant increase in the relative risk of precancerous cervical lesions such as abnormal Pap smears and cervical dysplasias has been associated with birth control use. This may be related to the false assumption that women on birth control are protected from sexually transmitted diseases such as herpes, syphilis, HIV, and HPV. Since sexually transmitted diseases are ever present in our society, particularly chlamydia and herpes, women of all ages need to protect themselves by having their partners use latex condoms. Remember that latex condoms are the *only* condoms effective against HIV. Have a few condoms on hand in case your partner forgets them. You are sleeping with every sexual contact that your partner has ever had.

MYTH: Birth control should not be taken by women over the age of thirty-five.

REALITY: As long as you are a non-smoker and do not have a personal or family history of one of the following: active liver disease, deep venous thrombosis (blood clot that frequently occurs in the deep veins of the legs), pulmonary embolus (blood clot in the lung), stroke, or breast cancer, birth control may be taken from a time a woman begins her menses until her menopausal years. In fact, birth control provides an excellent method of regulating the often erratic menstrual cycles in young women who may only experience a period every three to six months during the first few years after beginning their menses. Birth control pills, patches, and rings can also be used to treat acne, a common problem during both adolescence and perimenopause. Similarly, birth control may be used to normalize the often erratic and heavy menstrual flow that some women experience in their perimenopausal years.

MYTH: Birth control pills are expensive.

REALITY: A one-month supply of birth control pills costs between $10 and $50. This amounts to the price of a cup of coffee per day! Most insurance plans will pay for certain generic brands of birth control with a minimal copay and will pay for brand name birth control with a higher-tiered copay. If your particular brand is not covered by your insurance company and you have found that this is definitely the brand for you, ask your gynecologist to call in a "medical override" to your insurance carrier so that it will be covered on your plan. Most gynecologists stock their offices with an array of birth control samples, amply provided by pharmaceutical companies. These samples may help you to defray the costs of birth control if you must pay for it in cash. Finally, keep in mind the emotional strain, anxiety, and monetary cost of an unplanned pregnancy.

MYTH: Birth control causes significant weight gain.
REALITY: Birth control pills, rings ,and patches do not contain any calories; however, women fear that these contraceptives may adversely affect their metabolism, thereby causing them to gain weight. With the new classes of progestational agents that emerged in the 1990s (birth control pills contain two hormones, estrogen and progestin), the numbers of women reporting weight gain on birth control has declined significantly. Most pharmaceutical companies that produce pills, rings, and patches report a one to three pound weight gain over a year's time. Many patients crave carbohydrates while on the pill, patch, or ring. If this is happening to you, make sure that you have raw veggies and low-carb snacks available at all times.

MYTH: Birth control is unnecessary to prevent pregnancy in perimenopause (the years prior to menopause).
REALITY: Next to unmarried women under the age of twenty-five, the second highest number of unintended pregnancies occur in women over the age of forty. The perimenopausal period encompasses the stage in a woman's life when ovarian function is slowly failing. All women are born with a finite number of follicles (eggs), about 400. By the average age of fifty-two in this country, this number is depleted. This may lead to hot flashes and irregular menstrual cycles;

however, ovulation and consequent pregnancy may ensue if adequate contraception is not used.

Besides preventing pregnancy, birth control pills, patches, rings, and the intrauterine device serve as effective treatment for hot flashes, vaginal dryness, moodiness, and irritability often reported during the menopausal period. Even if you have had your tubes tied for contraception, birth control can help you with these symptoms as well. Once a woman has entered true menopause by either the cessation of menses on the pill-free days of her cycle or by a follicle stimulating hormone (FSH) blood test over thirty units, she can be safely changed over to hormone replacement therapy. On the other hand, I have seen two cases in which my patients started to menstruate after their FSH levels were over thirty units. One of them even became pregnant and miscarried. That is why it is important to have this FSH level rechecked if your menstrual cycles restart after stopping for a few months.

Furthermore, birth control pills, patches, and rings have been shown to increase HDL ("good" cholesterol) and may help to prevent heart disease.

MYTH: Birth control causes infertility.

REALITY: The average healthy woman between the ages of eighteen and thirty-five who discontinues birth control to conceive a pregnancy will do so within one year of stopping birth control. Within twenty-four months, more than 90 percent of previous birth control users become pregnant. If you are unable to achieve a pregnancy after one year off of the pill, you and your partner will benefit from an infertility workup, to search for the underlying causes. Typically, if you were started on birth control because you were not having periods or because your periods were irregular, you will continue to have the same problems when you stop taking the pill.

MYTH: Birth control can cause serious birth defects if a woman conceives while taking them.

REALITY: Studies have shown that children born to mothers who were taking birth control at the time of conception and even after conception had no increased rate of birth defects as compared to that found in the general population, a rate of 2 to 3 percent. In my own personal practice, the above has proven to be true.

MYTH: Birth control cannot be used while breastfeeding.

REALITY: Breastfeeding does **not** protect a woman from pregnancy. By the third month postpartum, 18 percent of women will have ovulated. Whereas estrogen and progesterone containing pills have been shown to decrease milk production and quality in the postpartum period and therefore should be avoided during breastfeeding, the progesterone only pill—or mini-pill—has no adverse effect on milk production, and provides effective contraception. It can be started immediately after delivery.

MYTH: A woman must menstruate every month.

REALITY: Birth control, since its inception, has been taken by women twenty-one days out of every month, with a week off for withdrawal bleeding. It was initially thought that this week of bleeding was necessary, as it mimicked a woman's natural menstrual cycle. However, as more and more women have entered the workforce, this week of bleeding has become nothing more than a nuisance. The menstrual cycle contributes to decreased productivity in the workplace, due to often unbearable cramps, headaches, dizziness, and nausea associated with menstrual bleeding.

Gynecologists for years have been prescribing continuous birth control so that women can skip their menses in order to attend events such as weddings or vacations. When birth control pills, patches, or rings are taken without a one-week break each month, a woman can miss a menstrual cycle for either one month or for consecutive months. Women may notice an astonishing reduction in bloating, menstrual migraine headaches, and other PMS symptoms.

How should continuous birth control be taken? Typically, a woman continues onto another birth control pill pack after she finishes her twenty-first active pill in the pack. The best type of pill to take for continuous therapy should be a pill that contains the same amount of estrogen and progesterone daily, e.g. Femcon®, Yasmin®, Orthocyclen®, and Loestrin®. I find that pills in which the progesterone levels increase weekly cause more breakthrough bleeding. Another form of contraception, the Nuvaring®, can be placed vaginally once a month to provide continuous contraception. Two continuous pills on the market are Seasonique®, which is taken for eighty-seven days straight, resulting in four periods each year, and Lybrel®, which is taken continuously all year long. The progesterone containing intrauterine device Mirena® induces amenorrhea, the cessation of menses, approximately three to six months after it is inserted.

The only side effect of continuous birth control is occasional breakthrough bleeding. I tell my patients that if bleeding persists for more than two days after doubling up on their birth control pills, they should stop the pill, bleed for one week, then restart a brand new pill pack. What is the downside to not having a menstrual cycle monthly? Absolutely nothing! The uterine lining is protected from overgrowing by a constant daily dose of two complementary hormones, estrogen and progesterone. What is the upside of continuous therapy? Think of all the money you will be saving on tampons, pads, and pain medication!

Birth control in the form of pills, patches, rings, and intrauterine devices (IUDs) is used by millions of women throughout the world for contraception. One type does not fit all, but if it works for you, you can reap the many non-contraceptive benefits of birth control through your perimenopausal years.

Ask your gynecologist or primary care provider for information on birth control at your next annual exam. The two of you can decide which birth control method is right for you.

Chapter 3

The Morning After

A patient once paged me at 3:00 AM to tell me that the condom that she and her boyfriend were using broke, and that she may have been ovulating. They were not prepared for an unintended pregnancy and wanted to know what they could do to prevent it.

Unintended pregnancies are on the rise in our country. There are approximately 3 million unintended pregnancies in the U.S. annually. Teenagers account for approximately 590,000 of these births, and 350,000 teenagers undergo abortions annually. Unplanned pregnancies could be avoided by educating the public about the safety and efficacy of the "morning after pill."

Emergency contraception is safe and effective if used in a timely manner. A woman must take two elevated doses of birth control pills within seventy-two hours of unprotected intercourse. These two doses are given twelve hours apart. This effective method—known as the "Yuzpe" regimen—has been available for years, just not widely publicized. The method is based on providing a hostile uterine environment with large doses of estrogen and progesterone so that an embryo cannot implant. Use of the morning after pill has been proven to reduce the risk of pregnancy by 75 percent.

Emergency contraception may be used for any of the following circumstances:

1. The condom breaks.
2. A woman misses more than two birth control pills in a month and has unprotected intercourse.
3. She has unprotected sex during her first month on birth control.
4. She is late for her Depoprovera® injection, which should be given every three months.
5. A rape occurs.
6. A diaphragm, cervical cap, or contraceptive sponge slips out of place.

The U.S. Food and Drug Administration announced that six brands of combined oral contraceptive pills are safe and effective for emergency contraception. These brands include: Ovral®, Lo-Ovral®, Levlen®, Nordette®, Tri-Levlen®, and Triphasil®. Two Ovral® pills need to be taken within seventy-two hours of unprotected intercourse, followed by two more Ovral® pills twelve hours later. For all of the remaining pills mentioned, four pills need to be taken immediately, followed by four pills twelve hours later.

My patients are often concerned about side effects of taking such a high dose of birth control. These effects include nausea and vomiting, which will cause them to be ineffective. I usually instruct my patients to take two of the four pills immediately, followed by two pills two hours later. They are then told to repeat this process in twelve hours.

I will often prescribe an anti-emetic such as Compazine® or Zofran® to combat the nausea.

Plan B, which consists of two pills of high-dose progestin taken twelve hours apart, is now available at certain pharmacies around the country without a prescription. It is usually well tolerated.

If the morning after pill fails to prevent the pregnancy, the literature shows that there is no increased risk for fetal anomalies.

If you would like more information about the morning after pill, call the Emergency Contraception Hotline at **1-800-584-9911** or access the Emergency Contraception Website at ***http://opr.princeton. edu/ec/.***

Chapter 4

Human Papillomavirus and Cervical Disease

"I want to be one less person affected by cervical cancer," states the young woman in the Merck campaign advertisement for the Gardasil® or human papillomavirus vaccine. So what does it mean if your doctor informs you that you have been exposed to **human papillomavirus** (HPV)? Your Pap smear may have been normal or it may have been abnormal. First of all, do not panic. You do not have cervical cancer or an incurable disease. However, you are going to need close follow-up so that the virus does not progressively invade your cervix.

Human papillomavirus (HPV) is a human virus. It comes in more than 100 different types. Approximately 40 percent of sexually active women **and men** carry the virus. It is extremely common. Men, fortunately, do not develop testicular or penile cancer from HPV; however, they can pass the sexually transmitted disease on to women through unprotected intercourse. I am often asked, "How long have

I had HPV?" Presently, there is no way to determine how long you have had HPV; therefore, any partner you have ever had may have been infected.

The most benign types are HPV #6 and #11. These are the causative agents of condyloma or warts. Both you and your sexual partner can develop warts. Warts need to be burned off with acid or frozen off with cryotherapy. (These can both be done in a doctor's office.) If you wish to treat yourself, your physician can prescribe an immunomodulator called Aldara® cream, which you can apply to the affected area every other day until the lesions disappear. Condyloma can reoccur, so it is important that you perform self-examinations regularly after treatment.

The high risk types of HPV are types 16, 18, 31, and 33. If you have been sexually exposed to these types of HPV, it may cause changes in your cervix, known as cervical dysplasia. Cervical dysplasia involves the way in which the nucleus of your cervical cells looks to a pathologist under a microscope.

Since a Pap smear is only a screening test for cervical cancer, you must undergo a follow-up colposcopy or examination of the cervix and vagina under a microscope, to see whether or not the human papillomavirus has infected your cervix. If the cervical biopsy returns low-grade dysplasia (LSIL), you will need close follow-ups with Pap smears every four months for one year. LSIL will resolve spontaneously in up to 85 percent of women within one year if you take a good multivitamin (I recommend a multivitamin with at least 400 micrograms of folic acid and Coenzyme Q10 100mg/day. Juice Plus® is also an excellent supplement (four capsules contain the equivalent of four servings of fruits and vegetables each day) to boost your immune system.

Human Papillomavirus and Cervical Dysplasia

If the biopsy shows a higher grade lesion on your cervix, known as high-grade dysplasia (HSIL), you will need to have a piece of your cervix removed under general anesthesia. This is called a cone biopsy of the cervix. A high-grade dysplasia has more of a tendency to progress to cervical cancer in five or more years than a low-grade dysplasia. Therefore, surgical intervention is necessary.

Occasionally, a cervical biopsy or cone biopsy pathology specimen will return with a diagnosis of invasive cervical cancer. This occurs in women who have not had a Pap smear in many years or failed to follow up an abnormal Pap smear in the past. If the cancer is localized to the cervix, a simple hysterectomy is curative. However, if the cancer has spread beyond the cervix, a radical hysterectomy, which involves removing the uterus, cervix, and tissue adjacent to the uterus, along with radiation therapy is necessary. Cervical cancer grows slowly. This is why it is so important to undergo annual Pap smears in order to find and treat cervical changes early.

Human papillomavirus will not affect your ability to become pregnant or to have a vaginal birth in the future. The virus is rarely transmitted to a fetus through the birth canal, unless a woman has extensive vulvar and vaginal warts at the time of delivery. The child may acquire esophageal or laryngeal papillomatosis or an infection of the throat or windpipe.

Merck Pharmaceutical Company launched their HPV vaccination (Gardisil®) in 2007, which has been approved by the FDA to be given to girls and women between the ages of twelve and twenty-six. This vaccination decreases a woman's lifetime risk of acquiring HPV types that cause condyloma (warts) and/or cervical dysplasia by approximately 90 percent. If a woman already has been diagnosed with

HPV, she still may be a candidate for the vaccination, under certain conditions. The vaccination is given in three intervals: at the time of the first visit, then two months later, and then four months later. The side effects of the vaccination have been proven to be minimal, and include a rash at the injection site and temporary fever.

Glaxo SmithKline Inc.'s newest vaccination called Cervarix® is presently under clinical trials and has yet to be approved by the Food and Drug Administration. The trials include women between the ages of ten and fifty-five. Once this vaccination is approved, women over the age of 26 will also have insurance coverage for the vaccine.

Most insurance companies are covering the vaccination, which costs roughly $150 per injection. Speak to your gynecologist about receiving the vaccination, even if you do not fall into the age category for which the FDA approved it. You could be one less woman affected by HPV!

Chapter 5

Herpes: More Common than You Think

A seventy-three-year-old patient presents with blisters on her vulva for the first time in her life. A twenty-three-year-old patient tells me that the sores on her vulva hurt so badly that she cannot urinate. An eighty-three-year-old patient has been complaining of burning upon urination for weeks, and has been treated for a urinary tract infection twice with no relief. A forty-five-year-old patient notices stinging around her rectum when she has a bowel movement. An eighteen-year-old woman presents with a cold sore. What do all of these women have in common? Herpes.

Herpes is one of the most common yet misdiagnosed sexually transmitted diseases in the United States. Although 50 million men and women have been diagnosed with herpes, countless others harbor the disease asymptomatically. Even if a woman presents with an active herpes lesion, a culture performed on a the site may return negative for the disease. That is why it is especially important to undergo blood testing. Two tests should be performed, an HSV I

IgG antibody test and an HSV II IgG antibody test. These two tests will show if you have had an infection in the past and now harbor herpes asymptomatically. I am commonly asked by patients, "How long have I had this?" and "Who do you think gave this to me?" Unfortunately, unless it is a very new infection or a first outbreak, it is nearly impossible to determine how long a patient has had herpes. Most of my patients who are routinely tested with blood work that returns positive have never even had an oubreak.

The most common herpes viruses are herpes simplex virus type 1 (HSV-1) and herpes simplex virus type 2 (HSV-2). Usually HSV-1 causes cold sores, while HSV-2 causes lesions below the waist, causing genital and perirectal herpes. But be aware that both HSV-1 and HSV-2 viruses can cause herpes outbreaks in either area. For instance, having oral sex with an active cold sore can spread HSV-1 to the genitals of your partner. Other common herpes infections include chicken pox and shingles, which are caused by the herpes zoster virus. Transmission is caused by close oral, anal, or genital contact, including intercourse, masturbation, kissing, or any direct skin-to-skin contact that allows for the transfer of bodily fluids. A person is considered contagious when symptoms that precede an outbreak such as itching and burning, active sores, and/or healing lesions are present.

Herpes is potentially contagious even when there are no symptoms. That is, a person who has genital herpes is potentially always shedding active virus. Approximately one in six members of the general infected population is thought to shed active virus occasionally without symptoms.

Some people do not get typical blister-like sores, but harbor active virus in their saliva, or vaginal or penile secretions, and can shed the virus without knowing they have herpes. Lesions can occur deep inside the vagina and the cervix, where they cannot be seen or felt, but can readily transmit the virus. An uninfected individual has about a 75 percent chance of contracting herpes during intimate contact with someone actively shedding virus.

Auto-inoculation occurs when an infected individual spreads the virus to other parts of his or her body by touching an area that is shedding virus and then touching, scratching, or rubbing another susceptible part of the body. Towels are especially conducive to this, and can also transmit the herpes virus to members of a family. That is why it is so important to not share toothbrushes and towels, and to line the toilet seat if one has a known herpes outbreak.

Treatment for active herpes involves acyclovir twice per day for seven days or Valtrex® twice per day for three days. This is not a cure for the virus, but it will allow the symptoms to abate more rapidly. For patients who have more than three outbreaks per year, I suggest continuous acyclovir or Valtrex® therapy. This involves taking a daily pill to suppress the virus. This can stop outbreaks altogether, with minimal side effects. Adverse side effects that patients can expect on antiviral therapy include headache, nasal congestion, and upper respiratory tract infection. In practice, I have never seen one of these side effects in patients on continuous therapy.

Should a woman who is trying to become pregnant or already is pregnant concern herself with herpes? The answer is yes. There is a 30 to 40 percent transmission rate of herpes to the newborn with a first herpes episode at the time of delivery. The transmission rate falls to 4 percent with a recurrent outbreak. Either way, the patient must undergo a cesarean section to lessen the viral load that is transmitted to the newborn. Infected newborns may have mild symptoms at first, such as a low-grade fever, poor feeding, or one or more small skin lesions. This may happen two to twelve days after exposure. Newborns can then become very ill, with high fevers, seizures, and lethargy (lack of energy). To prevent these infections from occurring at the time of delivery, I place my patient on either acyclovir or Valtrex® twice a day at the thirty-sixth week of pregnancy until delivery. Then I continue this therapy until six weeks postpartum. These antiviral therapies are both safe to use while breastfeeding.

Herpes infections can often be disguised as one of many other common gynecologic infections, such as a urinary tract infection, vaginitis, and yeast infections. Presenting symptoms may include itching, burning, redness, discharge, painful urination, and urinary urgency and frequency. If any of these symptoms become persistent despite multiple therapies such as creams or antibiotics, it is advisable to undergo herpes testing. Although you will carry this virus with you for the rest of your life, it can be controlled with proper diet and exercise to boost the immune system, and by antiviral therapy if outbreaks become recurrent.

References: Centers for Disease Control and Prevention Web site. *www.cdc.gov*, August 10, 2006.

Chapter 6

Over-the-counter Yeast Medication: Cure or Culprit?

Over-the-counter antifungal medications for the treatment of vulvovaginal candidiasis, more commonly known as a "yeast infection," entered the market in the early 1990s. By 1995, these products accounted for nearly 60 percent of the 482 million dollars per year spent on over-the-counter feminine healthcare products. By the year 2000, billions of dollars were spent on these products.

It has been estimated that of the millions of women who buy over-the-counter antifungal medications, fewer than 30 percent of these women actually have a true yeast infection that would be culture positive in a physician's office.

In a review of 220 women who were seen by a gynecologist for vaginal irritation, 75 percent of these presented with excessive vaginal discharge. Vaginal specimens from all 220 women were cultured for yeast, and only **11 PERCENT** had a positive culture!

So why are so many women running to supermarkets and drugstores to treat an infection that they probably do not have? They are looking for a quick fix to their problem, one that does not involve taking time off from work and visiting a doctor's office, which often disrupts their daily schedules.

In fact, as many as 75 percent of all women will experience at least one episode of yeast in their lifetime. More than 45 percent of women will experience two or more episodes each year. Diabetics and other women with immunodeficiencies may experience even more. The problem lies in the multitude of other vaginal infections and conditions with which a woman may confuse a yeast infection.

The important point to stress is that not every woman with an abnormal vaginal discharge, itching, or burning has a yeast infection. It may be a serious condition requiring medication attention.

Factors that predispose a woman to develop yeast infections include antibiotic use, pregnancy, diabetes, and chronic medical conditions in which patients use high doses of steroids, such as asthma, lupus, and arthritis.

The predominant symptom of a vaginal yeast infection is intense itching and burning. The discharge is usually white and may have the appearance of cottage cheese. However, the discharge may also be yellow or green. It is usually odorless. The diagnosis of the infection is established by performing a microscopic evaluation of the discharge or by vaginal culture, which may take twenty-four to forty-eight hours to process.

A more common infection, which accounts for approximately 50 percent of all gyn office visits for vaginitis, is bacterial vaginosis. This infection is caused by an overgrowth of a bacterium known as gardnarella. Women with bacterial vaginosis present with an unpleasant vaginal odor that they describe as "fishy." The discharge color is usually thin and gray-white in appearance. This particular infection has been implicated in a number of serious consequences if left untreated, such as pelvic inflammatory disease (infection of the uterus, cervix, and fallopian tubes, which may lead to infertility), and premature labor and rupture of membranes during pregnancy.

Besides bacterial vaginosis, other sexually transmitted diseases such as trichomonas, chlamydia, gonorrhea, and herpes may present with a vaginal discharge and irritation. If left untreated or improperly treated, these organisms can have devastating effects on the female reproductive tract.

In menopausal women, the usual culprit of vaginal irritation is atrophic vaginitis or simply put, a lack of estrogen associated with menopause. This condition can be easily treated, once properly diagnosed, with either oral estrogen or topically treated with vaginal estrogen cream or tablets. Many of these women have treated themselves with prescription and over-the-counter medications for infections that they simply do not have, which may then cause an allergic reaction and worsen the itching or burning.

Before heading for the over-the-counter remedy aisle in your local pharmacy, assess yourself. Do you have the symptoms of a yeast infection or could it be something else? Your doctor's office is just a phone call away, and could save you both time and money.

Chapter 7

The Ovarian Cyst

Twenty-eight-year-old Shelly presents to my office with pelvic pain. Her pain is located in the left lower quadrant of her abdomen and is consistent. She denies nausea, vomiting, diarrhea, pain with urination, and fever. I perform a pelvic exam and determine that her pain is coming from her left ovary. A pelvic ultrasound confirms that there is a three centimeter clear fluid-filled cyst in her left ovary.

Pelvic pain is a common reason for gynecology appointments. However, ovarian cysts are just one of a multitude of underlying physiological problems that can cause pelvic pain.

I first need to rule out kidney stones, constipation, food poisoning or other gastrointestinal disturbances, gallstones, appendicitis, pancreatitis, and muscle pulls or tears due to strenuous exercise or heavy lifting. I can usually eliminate most of these problems with a careful history. I will ask my patients about the location, duration, severity, and radiation of the pain. Blood work, including a white blood cell count, hematocrit, liver function tests, lipase and amylase will then be drawn, and a urine culture will be sent. She or he will then send you for one of the following imaging tests: CAT scan, MRI, ultrasound, or X-ray.

By interviewing and examining Shelly, I determined that the cause of her pain is indeed an ovarian cyst. How did she develop this? The ovaries produce cyst-like structures called follicles each month. Follicles produce the hormones estrogen and progesterone, and release an egg when you ovulate.

Sometimes a normal monthly follicle just keeps growing. When that happens, it becomes known as a functional cyst. There are two types of functional cysts:

- **Follicular cyst.** Around the midpoint of your menstrual cycle, your brain's pituitary gland releases a surge of luteinizing hormone (LH), which signals the follicle holding your egg to release it. When all goes well, the egg is released from its follicle, is picked up by the fallopian tube, and then travels to the uterus.

  Follicular cysts form when the LH surge fails to occur, resulting in a follicle that fails to release its egg. It instead grows and turns into a cyst. Follicular cysts rarely cause pain, and often disappear within two or three menstrual cycles.

- **Corpus luteum cyst.** When LH does surge and your egg is released, the ruptured follicle begins producing large quantities of estrogen and progesterone in preparation for conception. This changed follicle is now called the corpus luteum. At times, the opening of the follicle where the egg is released fails to close, and fluid accumulates inside the follicle, causing the corpus luteum to expand into a cyst.

Although this cyst usually disappears on its own in a few weeks, it can grow to the size of an orange and has the potential to bleed into itself or twist the ovary, causing pelvic or abdominal pain. If it fills with blood, the cyst may rupture, causing internal bleeding and sudden, sharp pain.

What are some of the symptoms of ovarian cysts?

- Menstrual irregularities
- Pelvic pain — a constant or intermittent dull ache that may radiate to your lower back and thighs
- Pelvic pain during intercourse (dyspareunia)
- Pain during bowel movements or pressure on your bowels
- Nausea, vomiting, or breast tenderness similar to that experienced during pregnancy
- Fullness or heaviness in your abdomen
- Pressure on your rectum or bladder—difficulty emptying your bladder completely

The following three types of ovarian cysts are less common than the functional ovarian cysts; however, I am seeing more and more of these in women both young and old. These cystic masses may appear to be malignant on a CAT scan or ultrasound, and may require surgical exploration for a diagnosis.

- **Cystadenomas.** These cysts develop from ovarian tissue and may be filled with a watery liquid (serous) or a mucous (mucinous) material. I have seen these cysts as large as twenty-eight centimeters, the size of a seven month old fetus. The removal of these cysts usually will require the removal of the entire ovary and/or fallopian tube.

- **Dermoid cysts.** These cysts may contain body tissue such as hair, skin, nails, fat, and teeth, because they form from cells that produce human eggs. It is as if fetal tissue has begun to grow without the egg being fertilized. Rarely malignant, these cysts can become large and cause painful twisting or torsion of the ovary.
- **Endometriomas.** These cysts develop as a result of endometriosis, a condition in which uterine cells grow outside your uterus. Some of that tissue may invade your ovary and grow within it. These cysts are often referred to as "chocolate" cysts because of the thick brown fluid that they contain.

What is polycystic ovary syndrome?

Polycystic ovary syndrome (PCOS) is defined by the National Institutes of Health as hyperandrogenism (elevation of male hormones such as testosterone and androstenedione) and chronic anovulation. This syndrome occurs when a woman has a reverse ratio of pituitary hormones known as follicle-stimulating hormone (FSH) and leutenizing hormone (LH), with LH greater than FSH. When this occurs, women do not ovulate because ovarian follicles are not stimulated to grow, and a large number of small follicular cysts develop in their ovaries, which may look like a "string of pearls" on ultrasound examination. Women with this syndrome may be affected by obesity, irregular menstrual cycles, or no cycles at all (amenorrhea), acne and/or increased facial and body hair, and trouble conceiving a pregnancy. Treatment for PCOS includes weight loss, birth control pills, patches, or rings, and metformin, a diabetic drug that helps sensitize the body's cells to insulin. PCOS patients, particularly those who are overweight or obese, have been found to be resistant to insulin. This may lead to overt diabetes and possible heart disease in the future. The fertility drug clomiphene citrate has been used for many years to help women with PCOS to ovulate.

What is the treatment for ovarian cysts?

Treatment depends on your age, the type and size of your cyst, and your symptoms. Your doctor may suggest:

- **Wait and see.** You can wait and be re-examined in three months if you are in your reproductive years, you have no symptoms, and an ultrasound shows you have a simple, fluid-filled cyst. Your doctor will likely recommend that you get follow-up pelvic ultrasounds at periodic intervals to see if your cyst has changed in size.

  Menopausal women with clear fluid cysts less than five centimeters in diameter can be followed up in periodic intervals as well. These patients should undergo a **Doppler flow** of the cyst to rule out cancer. The Doppler flow tells the physician if there is significant blood flow to the cyst, often heralding a cancerous or precancerous lesion in a menopausal woman.

- **Birth control.** Your doctor may recommend the birth control pill, patch, or ring to reduce the chance of new cysts developing in future menstrual cycles. Contraceptives offer the added benefit of significantly reducing your risk of ovarian cancer—the risk decreases the longer you take birth control pills.

- **Surgery.** You may need to undergo a surgical procedure if the cyst grows or causes more pain.

  Some cysts can be removed without removing the ovary, in a procedure known as a cystectomy. This can be performed either laparoscopically with minimal incisions or through an open laparotomy, which involves either a "bikini cut" or a vertical incision from your pubic bone to your belly button. Your doctor may also suggest removing the affected ovary and leaving the other intact in a procedure known as oophorectomy. Both procedures may allow you to maintain your fertility if you're still in your childbearing years. Leaving at least one ovary intact also has the benefit of maintaining a source of estrogen production.

If a cystic mass is malignant, you will need to undergo a hysterectomy, removal of your ovaries and fallopian tubes, and a surgical staging procedure usually performed by a gynecologic oncologist. A general gynecologist may insufficiently stage an ovarian cancer, and then a re-operation needs to be performed to accurately determine the course of treatment.

My patients often ask me, "Should I take the Cancer Antigen 125 (CA 125) blood test to see if I am at risk for ovarian cancer?" A CA 125 examines the blood for an antigen that is produced by ovarian cancer and has been effectively used to monitor the progression and regression of ovarian cancer. Unfortunately, there are many other conditions such as pregnancy, menstruation, endometriosis, heart, liver, lung, and colon diseases that may also elevate a CA 125 level, making this test very nonspecific for ovarian cancer.

Laboratory Corporation of America® launched an ovarian cancer screening test, Ovasure™, in June 2008. This blood test uses six biomarkers for ovarian cancer that can discriminate between women who have the disease and women who do not. Research done at Yale University showed that the test was highly specific (those who were negative for the six biomarkers had a very high chance of *not* having the disease) and highly sensitive as well (those who are positive for the six markers had a very high chance of having the disease). This test is not covered by insurance plans, Medicare, or Medicaid, and costs between $250 and $300. The American Cancer Society estimates that 22,000 women will be diagnosed with ovarian cancer in 2008, and more than 15,000 lives will be claimed by the disease because it is usually diagnosed in an advanced stage when the cancer has spread. Ovasure™ will help to decrease these numbers, particularly in women who have a family history of the disease.

Routine pelvic examinations help ensure that changes in your ovaries are diagnosed as early as possible. Do not ignore symptoms that persist for more than two weeks, particularly if it involves pain that prevents you from accomplishing your daily activities. A simple diagnostic test can tell both you and your doctor what organ is causing the pain.

Reference: American Cancer Society. *Cancer Facts & Figures 2008*. Atlanta, Ga.: American Cancer Society, 2008.

Chapter 8

I Found a Lump in My Breast

Helen, a forty-three-year-old patient, comes to my office complaining of a lump in her breast that she feels has gotten larger over the past three months. Her mammogram one year prior to her visit was normal, and she has no family history of breast cancer. Helen is sure that she has breast cancer and urges me to send her to a breast surgeon for an immediate mastectomy! Instead, I perform a needle aspiration (fluid withdrawal) under ultrasound guidance of the breast mass, and the mass disappears.

After performing thousands of breast exams on women of all ages, I have come to the conclusion that not all breast masses are created equal. A sixty-two-year-old woman with a solid breast mass concerns me more than a thirty-two-year-old woman with multiple cystic breast masses. However, I do believe that all breast masses deserve an initial proper workup, including a bilateral breast mammogram and/or ultrasound.

The American Cancer Society recommends that all women receive a screening mammogram between the ages of thirty-five and forty. My patients often ask me why I do not send them routinely for mammograms before the age of forty. I inform them that mammography is not as sensitive in the dense breast of a younger woman for routine screenings. As a woman ages, her breasts are replaced by fatty tissue, which can be easily penetrated with X-rays. If you have a positive family history of breast cancer in a first-degree relative or are positive for the BRCA1 or BRCA2 gene (both confer a higher lifetime risk of breast cancer), routine screening mammograms often start as early as age thirty.

After age forty, all women should undergo yearly mammograms. If a suspicious nodule or calcification is noted on the mammogram, the radiologist will usually recommend a "spot compression view" and/or ultrasound of this lesion to get a better view of it. A solid mass will usually not compress, but a benign cyst will.

Remember, mammograms are not foolproof. There is a 15 percent false negative rate associated with mammography. This means that mammography may fail to pick up a cancer 15 percent of the time. I have had numerous instances in my career when a patient palpated a breast mass, the mammogram failed to pick it up, and a surgical biopsy revealed cancer. This is why I urge you to learn how to do a monthly breast exam with soapy hands in the shower after your period has ended. Please go to *www.breastcancer.org* and click on **"breast self exam"** to learn about a simple, quick exam that may save your life one day.

Digital mammography has become the standard of care for detecting breast lesions. It is a mammogram system in which the X-ray film is replaced by solid-state detectors that convert the X-ray into an electrical signal. The signals then produce an image of the breast that can be viewed on a computer system.

How does one prepare for a mammogram? First of all, do not schedule a mammogram for the week prior to your menses if your breasts are tender during this time. The best time to go for a mammogram is the week following your period.

The American Cancer Society recommends that you do not wear deodorant, talcum powder, or lotion under your arms during your mammogram. You should explain any symptoms or problems that you may have to the technologist performing the procedure. Please bring your old mammogram films with you to your visit, so that the radiologist has a comparison. Lastly, ask when and how you will be notified of the results.

Diagnostic centers and hospitals are required by law to notify patients of positive or negative results by mail. The technologist who is performing your exam does not have the authority to diagnose or discuss the results of your exam. Unfortunately, due to decreased reimbursements for mammography, a majority of radiologists neither examine patients prior to their mammograms nor discuss the results of a mammogram after it is read. My office is bombarded with phone calls about mammogram results. Note that it may take a few days for the radiologist to read your mammograms, as they are also comparing the present exam to your previous exams. Usually, the radiologist will call your physician shortly after he or she reads the mammogram if there is a suspicious lesion that needs immediate attention.

Magnetic resonance imaging (MRI) has been shown to detect cancers not visible on mammograms, but has long been regarded to have disadvantages. For example, although it is 27 to 36 percent more sensitive, it is less specific than mammography. As a result, MRI studies will have up to 5 percent more false positive results, which may result in more unnecessary biopsies. It is also a relatively expensive procedure ($1,000), and one that requires the intravenous injection of a radioactive agent that may have side effects. Some indications for using MRI for screening include:

- First-degree relative with breast cancer: mother, daughter, sister
- Patients with BRCA-1 or BRCA-2 tumor suppressor gene mutations
- Evaluation of women with breast implants
- History of previous lumpectomy or breast biopsy surgeries
- Very dense or scarred breast tissue

However, two studies published in 2007 demonstrated the strengths of MRI-based screening:

- In March 2007, an article published in the New England Journal of Medicine demonstrated that in 3.1 percent of patients with breast cancer, whose other breast was clinically and mammographically tumor-free, MRI could detect breast cancer.
- In August 2007, an article published in *The Lancet* compared MRI breast cancer screening to mammographic screening in 7,319 women. MRI screening was much more sensitive (97 percent in the MRI group vs. 56 percent in the mammography group) in recognizing early high-grade ductal carcinoma in situ (DCIS), the most important precursor of invasive carcinoma. The author of a comment published in the same issue of *The Lancet* concludes that "MRI outperforms mammography in tumor detection and diagnosis."

Your mammograms or MRI show a suspicious lesion and you have been referred to a breast specialist for a biopsy. What can you expect?

A needle biopsy of the breast is performed to remove suspicious cells using a hollow needle. The tissue is then examined under a microscope. **Image-guided biopsies** involve the use of an ultrasound or CAT scan to guide the surgeon or radiologist if the abnormal area of the breast is too small to palpate. In **stereotactic** breast biopsies, a special mammography machine using ionizing radiation helps guide the radiologist's needle to the site of the abnormal tissue. Stereotactic biopsies are performed when a mammogram shows a suspicious solid mass, a small cluster of calcium deposits known as microcalcifications, a distortion of the structure of the breast tissue, or a new mass or area of calcification at a previous surgery site.

If the breast biopsy returns with a benign diagnosis, you will be asked to undergo a diagnostic mammogram and ultrasound of that specific site in a short follow-up interval, between three and six months. If the biopsy returns with a malignant diagnosis, you will be referred to a breast surgeon, who will discuss your options of a lumpectomy or mastectomy based on the size and depth of the tumor, surgical staging, and lymph node involvement. Once the tumor and lymph nodes have been removed, you and your surgeon will discuss possible chemotherapy and/or radiation therapy, followed by an oral anti-estrogen such as Tamoxifen® or Femara® if the tumor is positive for estrogen and progesterone.

What are the risk factors for breast cancer and what can you do to prevent it?

Risk factors for breast cancer include:

1. Personal history of breast abnormalities

2. Beginning menses prior to the age of twelve
3. Age at first live birth (older first-time mothers have a higher risk)
4. Increased breast density
5. Use of hormone therapy in menopause
6. Having one or more first-degree relatives with breast cancer (sister, mother, father, daughter)
7. White women have more risk of being diagnosed with breast cancer than African-American women. However, African-American women are more likely to die of the disease.
8. Obesity

I cannot end a discussion on breast cancer risks without mentioning what I believe causes North American women to have the highest incidence of breast cancer in the world. Namely, a diet of meat, poultry, pork, and most recently discovered, alcoholic beverages. A majority of chickens, cows, and pigs in our country are injected with growth hormone to increase their muscle mass rapidly in order to make their way onto supermarket shelves and restaurant plates as quickly as possible. Growth hormone stimulates the production of estrogen in meat, milk products, and chicken, and this is what we are ingesting.

I have seen a huge surge in the number of young girls who are reaching puberty at younger ages, i.e. seven or eight years old. Their mothers bring them in to see me because they are menstruating while they are still in elementary school. I often find that these young girls have diets filled with fast food, which usually includes chicken and hamburgers. If your finances allow it, try to buy "greenwise" meats, poultry, and milk products in your grocery store. These products are produced without growth hormone, as it states on the label.

As for alcoholic beverages and increased breast cancer risk, a 2007 study by researchers at Kaiser Permanente in California analyzed data on the drinking habits of 70,033 women of various races and backgrounds. They were trying to determine whether the type of alcohol or just the amount a woman drinks impacts her breast cancer risk. Lead researcher, Dr. Yan Li, says they discovered that "it makes no difference if a woman drinks wine, beer, or liquor—it's the alcohol itself and the quantity consumed" that is critical. In fact, drinking three or more drinks a day may translate into an extra 5 percent of all women developing breast cancer as a result of heavy drinking.

So why are alcoholic beverages being implicated in breast cancer? It may be that alcohol, in large amounts, decreases blood levels of folic acid, a B vitamin that helps protect the body from breast cancer. More research needs to be done to test this hypothesis.

Pesticides such as DDT, dioxin, and atrazine are known as organochlorines because they are organic compounds containing chlorine bonded to carbon. These pesticides have also been implicated in breast cancer risk. Organochlorines are also produced in the manufacturing of herbicides, detergents, spermicidal foam or lubricants, petrochemicals such as polychlorinated biphenyls (PCBs), PVC plastics, and paper.

Organochlorines are not overtly toxic, but they mimic estrogen. Hormones function by attaching to cell receptors that are designed specifically for that hormone, and once connected, they trigger various chemical changes in the body. Natural estrogen, or estradiol, tends to be broken down relatively quickly by the body and then eliminated from the bloodstream. Chemicals that function like estrogen (called "xenoestrogens,") can bind to an estrogen receptor site, thereby preventing estradiol from binding and blocking its normal function. In contrast, natural plant xenoestrogens, like those occurring in broccoli, cabbage, and cauliflower, break down easily. Finally, organochlorines tend to stay in the body and remain active for a much longer time than natural estrogen, giving them the opportunity to do the body enormous harm.

What can we do to decrease the harm that xenoestrogens cause in our bodies? One way is to use the supplement DIM, (diindolylmethane), the active metabolite of indole-3-carbinol, a naturally occurring compound found in cruciferous vegetables such as broccoli and cabbage. DIM has been shown to have anti-cancer properties in both humans and animals. I tend to prescribe DIM for all of my breast cancer survivors and in my patients who take hormone replacement therapy and who have family histories of breast cancer.

Other ways to decrease organopesticides in our environment include:

- Reduce or eliminate use of plastic containers for food storage.
- Purchase unbleached coffee filters, paper, napkins, toilet tissue, tampons, etc. The Environmental Protection Agency has determined that using bleached coffee filters alone can result in a lifetime exposure to dioxin that exceeds acceptable risks.
- Use tampons and sanitary napkins made of organic cotton without chlorine. (The FDA detected dioxins and dozens of other harmful substances in tampons.)
- Do not use chlorine bleach for household cleaning or laundry. Instead, use hydrogen peroxide.
- Drink filtered or bottled water, not "city water" that contains chlorine.
- Do not use pesticides or herbicides.

- Use plant-derived alternatives to hormone replacement therapy.
- Decrease use of plastic products (their production releases chlorinated toxins into the environment).
- Use only natural underarm deodorants; avoid antiperspirants.
- Avoid animal foods that contain hormones, such as milk, chicken, beef, and pork. Avoid char-broiled or barbecued cooking.
- To counter free radicals, eat foods high in antioxidants (vitamins A, C, E, selenium, beta carotene), green leafy vegetables, kale, carrots, yams, sweet potatoes, citrus, nuts, broccoli, and cauliflower.
- Eat organically grown food.

Breast cancer will be responsible for more than 220,000 deaths in our country this year. Be proactive in preventing this disease by undergoing a routine breast exam, along with a routine mammogram, reporting any unusual breast lumps immediately, avoiding pesticides in the food you eat, eating less meat and poultry, and substituting fish and vegetables instead, and maintaining a healthy weight.

For more information about breast cancer, visit *www.nci.gov* and search for "breast cancer."

Chapter 9

Do I Really Need a Hysterectomy?

A forty-eight-year-old African-American schoolteacher and mother of three comes to see me for a consult. She tells me that her menstrual cycles have become heavier over the past two years, that her pants are feeling tighter, and that intercourse has become more painful. She presents me with an ultrasound report, which reveals that her uterine size is that of a large grapefruit. When she saw her gynecologist last year, she was told that her uterus was the size of a lemon.

What are my patient's options? Does she wait until menopause and do nothing? Does she undergo a total abdominal hysterectomy? Or does she have other options?

Gynecologists in the United States perform well over 600,000 hysterectomies each year. Patients who undergo hysterectomies usually present to their doctors with a fibroid uterus and the complaints of painful menses and heavy bleeding. With the advent of laparoscopy or minimally invasive surgery in the late 1970s and the rapid improvement of laparoscopic equipment and techniques over the years, women now have the option of removing the uterus with minimally invasive surgery. Instead of using a large bikini-cut incision, which can extend from one hip to the other, a gynecologist can now remove a uterus with just three small abdominal incisions. How does the surgeon remove a uterus that can be the size of a grapefruit or small melon through a one-centimeter incision? A technique known as morcellation uses a device that functions somewhat like an apple peeler. It cuts pieces of tissue into long, thin tubes, which can be removed through a small incision in the abdomen.

During a laparoscopic supracervical hysterectomy, the cervix is maintained, thereby preventing pelvic prolapse in the future and maintaining the plexus of nerves on the cervix, which are very important for sexual pleasure during intercourse. In a total laparoscopic hysterectomy, most of the surgery is performed through three small incisions; however, the surgeon can then remove the uterus and cervix vaginally. Patients who undergo these laparoscopic procedures are usually discharged from the hospital the following day and can return to work in one to two weeks. I have had a schoolteacher undergo a laparoscopic hysterectomy on Friday and return to the classroom the following Monday without any physical restrictions.

My patients often cannot afford to take two to six weeks off from work or simply wish to avoid the risks of major surgery? For these women, uterine artery embolization (UAE) is a viable option.

UAE involves the injection of the uterine arteries (which are the main blood supply to the uterus) with small, inert particles by an interventional radiologist. This procedure is typically performed in a hospital setting so that the patient can be admitted overnight for pain management. UAE is contraindicated in women who wish to maintain their fertility as the decrease in blood supply to the uterus could adversely affect a pregnancy. Conversely, UAE should not be used as contraception, as women can and have become pregnant after this procedure.

By eliminating half of the blood supply to the uterus, UAE allows the size of the uterus and fibroids to shrink by up to 50 percent in the first year following the procedure. This is associated with a significant reduction in bleeding and pain. Approximately 15 percent of patients undergoing UAE will need a hysterectomy for persistent symptoms.

If I determine that a patient's fibroids are inside the endometrial cavity (uterine lining) and not in the walls of the uterus, I will offer the patient a hysteroscopic vaginal myomectomy. This procedure involves entering the uterine cavity with a hysteroscope, which allows the surgeon to see inside the uterus. The fibroid can then be excised from the endometrial cavity and removed vaginally. This simple outpatient procedure allows the patient to return to work the following day without any abdominal scars.

Five Food and Drug Administration approved devices have been developed over the past ten years to surgically eliminate the lining of the uterus and either eliminate or decrease the amount of endometrial tissue that a woman sheds each month. The Novasure® ablation involves a microwave device that burns out the lining of the uterus, the Thermachoice® balloon ablation uses a balloon to do the same thing, and Her Option® uses a cold electrode to freeze the lining of the uterus. Hydro ThermAblator® circulates heated saline fluid inside the uterus and ablates the uterine cavity over ten minutes time. Microwave endometrial ablation (MEA®) uses microwave energy to heat the endometrium, using a small applicator that is moved from side to side in the uterus.

All five of these procedures result in scarring of the endometrial cavity. My patients are forewarned that childbearing should be completed prior to undergoing any one of these procedures. If pregnancy were to occur, the placenta may stick to the uterine wall after delivery of the baby, resulting in a hysterectomy at the time of birth and possible hemorrhage. I often combine a laparoscopic bilateral tubal ligation with a uterine ablation in order to prevent future pregnancies.

Lastly, a relatively new procedure known as magnetic resonance guided focused ultrasound (MRgFUS) was approved by the FDA in October 2004 as the first non-invasive treatment for uterine fibroids. MRgFUS uses highly focused ultrasound to locate the fibroid and then ablate it with heat and with pinpoint precision. The procedure lasts a few hours, can be performed in an outpatient setting, has minimal post-procedure pain, and allows the patient to return to normal activities almost immediately. The disadvantages of this procedure are that it often requires up to four hours, and it is not intended to treat large or multiple fibroids. Similar to the contraindications with uterine artery embolization, women who wish to become pregnant should not undergo this procedure.

MRgFUS is offered in multiple locations around the United States. It is a costly procedure because it uses a specialized MRI machine. There is limited third-party payment for the procedure. Prices for the procedure range from $10,000 to $20,000 per session.

Women with symptomatic fibroids and other causes of dysfunctional uterine bleeding have numerous options these days. No longer does a woman need to undergo major surgery with its associated costs, recovery, and time away from work and family. Speak with your gynecologist about your options and determine which procedure is right for you.

Chapter 10

Sometimes I Lose Urine

A fifty-two-year-old patient came to see me. She had delivered three children vaginally, and began to leak urine when she coughed or laughed since the birth of her last child. Now the leakage was becoming so bad that she had to wear a sanitary napkin every day. I asked her why she had not told her former gynecologist about this. She replied, "I thought that this was part of the aging process, and I was too embarrassed to talk about it."

Urinary incontinence affects 10 to 25 percent of women under the age of sixty-five, and 15 to 30 percent of women older than sixty years of age. More than 50 percent of nursing home patients suffer from incontinence, which is often the source of bed sores, sepsis from undiagnosed and prolonged urinary tract infections, and even death from these infections.

There are three types of urinary incontinence. The first, known as **urge incontinence,** occurs because the bladder muscle, known as the detrusor, is unstable and contracts unexpectedly. This may be the result of damage from childbirth, a lack of estrogen, or secondary to an underlying illness such as diabetes, multiple sclerosis, or spinal injury.

The second type of incontinence, **stress urinary incontinence,** usually occurs in women who have delivered one or more children vaginally. The pelvic floor, which includes a set of muscles and ligaments, supports the bladder, urethra, uterus, and rectum. After childbearing, the pelvic floor relaxes and loses some of these strong supports. As a result, a woman may experience the sensation of something dropping or falling from the vagina when she strains. This may be the uterus, bladder, rectum, or vagina. If a woman has had a previous hysterectomy, the vagina may fall. This patient will present to my office with the complaint of a "ball" coming out of the vagina, which makes walking difficult.

Pelvic floor relaxation leads to stress urinary incontinence because the angle between the urethra (urinary outflow tract) and bladder changes. It is this angle that helps to retain urine when a woman coughs, strains, or jumps. When the angle changes with pelvic relaxation, urine leaks when the bladder is placed under abdominal pressure.

Both stress and urge incontinence can occur together. This is called **mixed urinary incontinence.**

The third type of urinary incontinence, **overflow incontinence,** occurs because the bladder cannot completely empty itself. This leads to a steady leakage of small amounts of urine. This type of incontinence is mostly seen in nursing home patients and patients with neurological problems.

The diagnosis of incontinence is based upon a medical history taken in either a gynecologist's or an urologist's office. The doctor will ask you a series of questions regarding your voiding habits and your medical history. You will then be asked to prepare a twenty-four hour voiding diary. In this diary, you will record when and how much fluid you drank throughout the day. You will then record when you voided and how much you voided. Lastly, you will be asked to record when and if you felt a strong urge to void or when you lost urine throughout the day.

Most urologists will perform an in-office cystoscopy, which involves placing a small cystoscope into the bladder and visualizing the bladder opening, neck, and the inside of the bladder. A sterile urine specimen is then taken and also measured for a post-void residual to determine if you are completely emptying your bladder. The specimen is sent to the lab for evaluation of infection and/or cancer.

Cystometry involves measuring the bladder pressure and urethral pressure, both at rest and under the stress of bearing down. This procedure is also performed in a doctor's office without anesthesia. Probes are placed in both the urethra and rectum, and the bladder is slowly filled with room temperature fluid. The physician can tell what type of incontinence the patient has by using this procedure.

After the appropriate diagnosis has been made, treatment options can be offered. I initially treat both urge and stress incontinence medically. There are a variety of medications on the market that prohibit bladder spasms and cause bladder relaxation, to decrease the number of voids per day. I usually begin to treat urinary incontinence in the menopausal woman with hormone replacement therapy. Topical estrogen given vaginally helps to rejuvenate the bladder and urethra after a woman reaches menopause. This may actually help to prevent urinary incontinence.

Kegel's exercises have been a mainstay in first line non-medical treatment of stress incontinence. Kegel's exercises involve strengthening the pelvic floor muscles which have become lax secondary to childbearing or lack of estrogen. I usually instruct my patients to practice tightening their pelvic floor muscles by placing two fingers or a tampon applicator into the vagina and then squeezing the vaginal muscles over the item. Vaginal cones may be more effective and can be ordered by your gynecologist.

If medical therapy or exercise fails to improve urinary incontinence, surgical therapy can be offered only in the case of **stress urinary incontinence.** These procedures are bladder neck suspensions. They can be performed by a gynecologist experienced in urology or an urologist in an outpatient center. These quick outpatient procedures are performed vaginally with hypoallergenic mesh or tape. The mesh or tape forms a hammock under the urethra so that when the patient coughs or sneezes, the urethral angle with the bladder barely changes, resulting in continence. Some of the risks of the procedures include bleeding, infection, and expulsion of the tape or mesh. Rarely is a patient discharged with a catheter; however, if this occurs due to the inability to urinate after the procedure, it is usually removed within three to five days in the doctor's office.

Urinary incontinence is a common problem affecting millions of women in every age group. Incontinence does not have to be an awkward and embarrassing problem. It can be easily treated with simple medical therapy and exercise or with an outpatient procedure. You just have to ask!

Chapter 11

Menopausal Bleeding

I received a frantic call from a sixty-year-old patient named Ellen. Ellen had gone through menopause at the age of fifty-five without a problem and had awakened this morning to find her underwear stained with blood. She was not taking hormone replacement therapy, nor did she have a family history of gynecologic cancer. I asked her about her own gynecological history, and she denied any history of abnormal menstrual cycles in the past, as well as polyps or fibroids in her uterus. Was she at risk for uterine cancer?

Menopausal bleeding often causes anxiety because of its association with uterine cancer. Only 5 to 10 percent of women with menopausal bleeding will have biopsy-proven cancer. The majority of these women are bleeding due to an atrophic or thinned-out endometrial lining (lining of the uterus).

The first step in the work-up for menopausal bleeding is a pelvic or transvaginal ultrasound, in order to measure the lining of the uterus. If the uterine lining is five millimeters or less, both patient and physician can be reassured that the problem causing the bleeding is not cancerous. If the lining is greater than five millimeters, the patient will undergo an in-office endometrial biopsy of the uterus or an outpatient procedure known as a hysteroscopy (viewing of the inside of the uterus with a hollow chambered telescope). Women who take hormone replacement therapy often have thickened endometrial linings on ultrasound. This often leads to an exorbitant number of unnecessary biopsies. I rarely perform pelvic ultrasounds on my patients who have only been on hormone replacement therapy for less than six months. Monthly bleeding is usually normal as the unestrogenized uterus adapts to hormone therapy.

An in-office biopsy can be a painful procedure. I have my patients prepare by taking two ibuprofen one hour prior to the procedure, to avoid cramping afterward. Please forewarn your gynecologist if you are taking blood thinners or aspirin, which may cause excessive bleeding, or if you need prophylactic antibiotics for a heart condition or prosthetic joint. The procedure usually takes about five minutes and involves one to three passes of a tiny catheter into the uterine cavity. The tissue removed is then sent to a pathologist. The results return in approximately one week, depending on the particular laboratory.

When a diagnosis of endometrial hyperplasia (overgrowth of the uterine lining) or endometrial hyperplasia with atypia (abnormal appearing cells) is made on biopsy, the patient merely needs progesterone given orally to thin down the lining of the uterus. Endometrial hyperplasia is usually caused by an overabundance of estrogen, either given to the patient in the form of hormone replacement therapy or caused by the woman's own fat cell production of estrone, one of three types of estrogen, which stimulates the uterine lining. Consequently, obesity is the number-one risk factor for uterine cancer. Tamoxifen®, a common oral chemotherapeutic agent used to prevent breast cancer recurrence, frequently causes postmenopausal bleeding and increases a woman's chance of uterine cancer twofold. My patients who take Tamoxifen® undergo yearly pelvic ultrasounds. Typical findings on ultrasound include uterine polyps and endometrial hyperplasia, which can both be treated with a simple outpatient procedure.

Women with simple endometrial hyperplasia are treated with three months of a progestational agent such as medroxyprogesterone or norethindrone. These agents thin down the excess tissue, which is then shed by the uterus. The uterine lining is then re-biopsied after this three month period, to ensure that the tissue is normal. If the tissue remains abnormal, I will then proceed with a hysteroscopy combined with a dilatation and curettage (D & C). I am able to look inside the uterus with a camera to see if there is any other reason for the bleeding such as polyps, fibroids, or cancer.

Postmenopausal bleeding does not have to be frightening if you know the facts. As long as the appropriate workup is done in a timely fashion, you can assure yourself a favorable outcome.

Chapter 12

Life in the Flash Lane: Bio-Identical Hormone Replacement Therapy

In recent years, Suzanne Somers has graced the pages of prominent magazines and newspapers, touting the benefits of bio-identical hormone replacement therapy (HRT). She has also written about it extensively in her book, *The Sexy Years*. What makes this sixty-year-old former star of *Three's Company* and breast cancer survivor look so young and vibrant? Ms. Somers credits her hormone therapy that her endocrinologist specially compounds for her.

While I applaud Ms. Somers for bringing hormone replacement therapy back into mainstream society after it was deemed unsafe by the flawed 2002 Women's Health Initiative Study, hormone replacement therapy is not for everyone. One must first weigh the risks and benefits of the treatment after an extensive work-up.

Is there a difference between synthetic HRT and bio-identical HRT? Yes, there is. Wyeth Pharmaceutical Company introduced a synthetic estrogen product in the 1960s that was derived from the urine of pregnant mares. You may know this commonly prescribed HRT as Premarin®.

This synthetic estrogen product was marketed as the fountain of youth for which menopausal women had been waiting decades. All menopausal women could benefit from this medication because it would restore a woman's vitality and sex drive after she stopped menstruating.

Unfortunately, a large number of women taking Premarin® developed uterine cancer because, as we now know, unopposed estrogen stimulates the uterine lining unless it is opposed by progesterone. Wyeth soon after combined the popular Premarin® with medroxyprogesterone (MPA), a synthetic progestin, and marketed their product as Prempro®. Progestin is **not** a bio-identical hormone. This is not the same progesterone that the ovaries produce. It is a synthetic hormone that was created in a laboratory only to protect the uterine lining from overgrowing from the effects of estrogen replacement therapy.

For the past forty years, physicians had been prescribing this synthetic therapy and others like it for the relief of menopausal symptoms, until the results of the Wyeth-funded study on hormone replacement therapy known as the Women's Health Initiative (WHI) were published in the *New England Journal of Medicine* in 2002. This much publicized study found an increase in advanced breast cancer, stroke, and deep venous thrombosis (blood clot in the leg) if women took combined Prempro® for at least five years.

Since 2002, the WHI study has been scrutinized and re-studied. A huge flaw of this study was that the investigators studied women in their sixties, instead of their late forties and fifties, the average age of menopause in this country. Of course these women would have an increase in stroke, heart attacks, and blood clots, because their age and high blood pressure (38 percent of the study's participants were hypertensive) put them at risk for these adverse effects, even *without* taking hormone replacement therapy. Secondly, after five years, the investigators failed to find an increase in breast cancer occurrence in women who had only taken the estrogen alone, but an increase in breast cancer in those who had taken the combined estrogen and progestin therapy. What was the breast cancer culprit in this study? It appears that it was either the synthetic progestin, medroxyprogesterone, or MPA, in combination with estrogen. MPA has been known to cause bloating, vaginal bleeding, and an adverse change in a women's lipid profile, as it increases one's LDL or "bad" cholesterol. Could this progestin also stimulate breast cancer? So far the studies have been inconclusive. What the medical community did learn from this study was that women need to be carefully selected for hormone replacement therapy, and it should only be used for the minimum amount of time that it takes for a woman's symptoms to improve.

Bio-identical hormone replacement therapy (BHRT) was born in the 1980s. As a health food craze took over this country, women were looking for hormone replacement therapies that mimicked their body's own hormones. BHRT naturally replaces the hormones that the ovaries and adrenal glands produced before menopause. Perhaps the word "natural" should not be interchanged with "bio-identical" since "natural" connotes a product that is derived from nature, and bio-identical hormone therapy is prepared in a laboratory. It is true that the components of BHRT come from whole food products such as soy and yams; however, the estrogen and progesterone from these food sources are chemically altered, so they function just as they did in the ovary.

My patients often ask why they cannot purchase bio-identical HRT in a local pharmacy, using their insurance plans. The Food and Drug Administration cannot issue a patent on a naturally occurring substance such as bio-identical estradiol and progesterone, because it is identical to the hormones produced in the human ovary. Therefore, a large pharmaceutical company cannot mass produce this product. They are instead compounded by an ever-increasing number of compounding pharmacies, which are unregulated as to the content of the BHRT and of course, the pricing.

Before using BHRT, you will need to consult with your doctor—preferably a gynecologist or endocrinologist—and undergo either an extensive blood hormone work-up or saliva test. With this information in hand, your doctor will then prescribe a personalized formula designed to specifically meet your needs. Prior to receiving BHRT, every woman should undergo a physical exam, Pap smear, annual mammogram, and bi-annual bone density study or DEXA scan.

Bio-identical compounded hormones are prepared for maximal absorption. They may come in capsules, creams, sublingual drops or troches (lozenges), patches, vaginal creams, and suppositories. The products used for BHRT are plant based. They may contain any or all of the following hormones: estradiol, estriol, estrone, progesterone, dehydroepiandrosterone (DHEA) and testosterone.

It generally takes between two and four weeks for hormone levels to stabilize once therapy has been initiated. Hot flashes, moodiness, irritability, and sleep disturbances usually begin to subside in the first week of use.

The side effects that you may experience during the first six weeks of BHRT use include the following: breast tenderness, vaginal spotting or bleeding, nausea, headaches, and bloating. If bleeding is heavy and lasts more than three days, please call your doctor's office to schedule a visit. You may be asked to undergo a transvaginal ultrasound of the uterus to assess the uterine lining and/or undergo an in-office biopsy of the uterine lining, known as the endometrium.

What are the components of bio-identical hormone replacement therapy?

Progesterone

Progesterone is an important hormone for normal reproductive and menstrual function in reproductive years. It influences the strength and make-up of bone, blood vessels, heart, brain, and skin, among others. Progesterone is the building block for other hormones such as DHEA, cortisol, estrogen, and testosterone. It also plays a role in mental well-being, sugar balance, libido, thyroid, and adrenal function. It has been shown to increase bone density and decrease the risk of bone fracture, and can, by itself, be used to decrease hot flashes. Furthermore, progesterone is a natural diuretic that decreases bloating.

In the premenopausal woman, progesterone can be used to reduce the size of fibroids, thereby avoiding surgery, and can also help to reduce the size of endometrial implants and reduce pain in patients diagnosed with endometriosis. Progesterone has also been used extensively to prevent irritability, breast tenderness, bloating, and water-weight gain in the weeks preceding a woman's menses.

Estriol, Estradiol, Estrone

Estriol, estradiol, and estrone are produced by both the ovaries and in fat cells. Thus, an obese woman may enter menopause much later in life and have very heavy menstrual cycles.

Estriol is the estrogen that is produced in the least quantity by the ovaries. It is a weak form of estrogen that is used best on the vaginal mucosa. Preliminary research has shown that estriol may protect women against estrogen related cancers such as breast and uterine cancers.

In contrast, estradiol is the most abundant estrogen produced by the ovaries. It has the highest potency of all three types of estrogens. Its potency is twelve times that of estrone and eighty times that of estriol. Estradiol positively influences cardiovascular health, neurological function, bone density, vaginal health, and libido.

Estrone, on the other hand, becomes the primary estrogen produced in menopause, as the ovaries lose function. Estrone is synthesized not only in the adrenal glands but also through the conversion of another precursor hormone, androstendione, in adipose or fat tissue. Given that obesity has been proven to increase a woman's risk of developing breast and uterine cancer, estrone has been implicated as a causative agent, and therefore should not be compounded into bio-identical hormone therapy. Be aware that one of the most commonly compounded estrogens, known as Triest, typically contains 10 to 20 percent estrone.

Testosterone

Testosterone helps women maintain lean body mass, skin elasticity, bone density, and most importantly, libido or sex drive. This hormone is derived from progesterone and helps to increase the efficacy of the estrogens in decreasing hot flashes. Used as a cream two to three times per week, it can significantly boost libido after a few weeks of use. Unwanted side effects such as facial hair growth, hair loss, or acne should be reported to your doctor immediately.

Dehydroepiandrosterone

DHEA is a precursor to other hormones; it is produced by both the ovaries and the adrenal glands. DHEA gradually declines as a woman ages. It is important in the prevention of fatigue i.e. adrenal burnout, and also serves as an anti-inflammatory agent in conditions such as fibromyalgia, arthritis, lupus, and scleroderma. DHEA is best absorbed if taken by mouth.

Cortisol

Cortisol is the fight-or-flight hormone produced by the adrenal gland which sits atop the kidneys. It is responsible for storing fat, producing glucose from the liver in times of stress, the immune response, and blood pressure. During midlife, when most women are going through menopause, women experience high levels of stress and insomnia, often as a result of hot flashes and mood disturbances. Insomnia leads to high levels of ghrelin, the hunger hormone, and decreased levels of leptin, the fullness hormone, making insomniacs eat more than they would like. As a result of a lack of sleep and increased cortisol levels, the body packs all the calories from the absorbed foods that we eat into the abdomen and buttocks. Note that abdominal fat cells contain four times the cortisol receptors as the rest of the body. Now you can understand why menopausal patients often ask me why they cannot lose weight despite eating the same foods and exercising the same amount as they did before they went through menopause. Let's face it—after a restless night, does it really matter to you what you put into your mouth? Insomnia leads to cravings, particularly for carbohydrates, which in turn leads to weight gain.

Bio-identical HRT shares the same inherent risks as synthetic HRT, namely stroke, heart attack, blood clots, breast cancer, and uterine cancer. If given in a cream or patch form, BHRT will be absorbed directly into body tissues instead of entering the bloodstream and broken down by the liver. The above-mentioned risks are then substantially reduced by avoiding this "first pass" effect in the liver. Similarly, both cream and patch form do not interfere with the production of cholesterol in the liver, and in theory, should not have a negative impact on the circulatory system.

Should a woman take BHRT if she has been diagnosed with breast cancer or is a breast cancer survivor? What if she has a family history of breast cancer but has never had it herself? Most oncologists strictly forbid the use of any kind of hormone replacement therapy after breast cancer has been diagnosed.

I have a handful of breast cancer survivors in my practice who are on BHRT creams. All of these women are at least two years past their last chemotherapy or radiation therapy and have been deemed cured by mammograms and/or PET scan. Hormone replacement therapy has been labeled a causative agent of breast cancer. However, a synthetic form of estrogen replacement therapy, namely Premarin®, did not increase a woman's risk of breast cancer in the Women's Health Initiative Study. If a woman has a small estrogen or progesterone receptor-positive tumor growing undetected in her breast, it will most definitely be stimulated by exogenous hormone therapy. The good news is that women who develop breast cancer while taking HRT are usually diagnosed with a much earlier stage of breast cancer and have a better recovery and prognosis than women with breast cancer who are not taking HRT. In short, hormone replacement therapy—whether it is bio-identical or synthetic—**does not cause** breast cancer. Instead, **it may stimulate** the growth of a pre-existing cancer. I do believe that women suffering from hot flashes, vaginal dryness, sleeplessness, and decreased libido should not be denied hormone therapy because of a previous history of breast, ovarian, uterine, or even colon cancer.

Taking hormone replacement therapy is a personal choice that every woman must decide with the help of her physician. More than 500 of my patients are enjoying the benefits of bio-identical hormone replacement therapy with minimal side effects and only one known case of contained stage one breast cancer.

Please be sure that your physician has been trained in bio-identical hormone therapy, and that he or she is checking your hormone levels with either blood testing or saliva testing six to eight weeks after initiating HRT, and at least every year thereafter. It is possible to overdose patients on any kind of hormone therapy, and great care needs to be taken to keep a woman's hormones in correct balance without stimulating breast or uterine cancer. A common fallacy made popular in *The Sexy Years* is that women should have HRT-stimulated periods in menopause to simulate a natural menstrual cycle. This is absolutely incorrect! Any menopausal woman who has bleeding on HRT needs to be ruled out for uterine overgrowth, hyperplasia, or uterine cancer. If estrogen and progesterone levels are adequately balanced, a woman should never have a menstrual cycle on HRT.

The transition from premenopause to menopause does not have to be a rough one if hormone replacement therapy is used at the right time and in the correct dose. "Life in the flash lane" has gotten a lot better with bio-identical hormone replacement therapy.

Chapter 13

Make No Bones About It: Osteoporosis

A seventy-two-year-old thin white patient underwent a bone density study (DEXA) scan in my office, which showed a 5 percent decrease in the bone density of her hip and spine over the last two years, despite treatment with a biphosphonate, calcium, and vitamin D. Her mother sustained a hip fracture one year before her death. What are her options?

The above scenario has become all too common as record numbers of men and women are entering their golden years. Baby boomers are entering menopause in huge numbers as well. A record **17 billion dollars** will be spent this year on office visits, testing, hospitalizations, rehabilitation, and nursing home care for people suffering from osteoporosis. Now you can understand why prevention and early diagnosis are so important.

What is osteoporosis? It is a disease characterized by low bone mass and structural deformity, resulting in decreased bone strength and an increased risk of fracture. It is estimated that 44 million

Americans or 55 percent of the population over the age of fifty are affected. Ten million individuals are estimated to have osteoporosis, of which 8 million are women. An additional 34 million people are estimated to have osteopenia, the precursor to osteoporosis. Lastly, of the 300,000 hip fractures that are sustained by men and women in the United States each year, nearly 72,000 of these patients will die within a year of their fracture.

What are the risk factors for osteoporosis?

- Gender—Female
- Ethnicity—Caucasian and Asian
- Body Size—Small frame, low body weight (less than 125 pounds)
- Family history of osteoporosis
- Thyroid disease
- Hyperparathyroidism (overactive parathyroid gland)
- Gastrointestinal disorders that impair absorption of calcium and vitamin D
- Premature menopause either caused naturally or surgically by removal of the ovaries prior to menopause
- Cigarette smoking by decreasing estrogen production
- Excessive alcohol consumption, by increasing osteoblast activity and increasing the risk of falling
- High caffeine intake, by increasing loss of calcium in urine
- Inactive, sedentary lifestyle, by eliminating physical activity that stimulates bone remodeling
- Calcium and phosphorus deficiencies, which decrease formation of hydroxyapatite, the major mineral in bone

How is osteoporosis diagnosed?

Osteoporosis is diagnosed by a dual-energy X-ray absorptiometry or DEXA scan. A patient's hips and spine are scanned in an open machine in which one lies down on the back, fully clothed. A scanner in the form of a C-arm passes over the patient after the technologist positions the patient. The procedure lasts approximately fifteen minutes. The computer then generates a T-score. The T-score matches a patient with a thirty-year-old control match. This is the age in which bone density has reached a maximum. The lower the number or the more negative the number is, the worse the bone density is.

A T-score of greater than -1 is considered normal.
A T-score of -1 to -2.5 is considered osteopenia.
A T-score of less than -2.5 is considered osteoporosis.

I begin screening low risk patients at the age of fifty or the age of menopause, and then repeat the bone density study every two years. Women who are receiving therapy for severe osteoporosis should undergo bone density studies yearly.

When does one need treatment for osteoporosis?

The World Health Organization defines osteoporosis in menopausal women as a bone mineral density or BMD of greater than 2.5 standard deviations below the mean for young adult women (a T-score of < -2.5). Women should undergo treatment when they have T-scores of <-2.0 with no additional risk factors or BMD scores of <-1.5 with one or more additional risk factors, or when they have sustained a vertebral or hip fracture, regardless of BMD.

Non-pharmacological interventions to reduce fractures include:
- Weight-bearing exercise
- Muscle strengthening
- Fall prevention
- Avoidance of tobacco, soda, alcohol, and caffeine
- Balanced diet
- Adequate calcium and vitamin D intake

The recommended daily intake of calcium is 1,000 mg for premenopausal women and 1,200 mg for menopausal women. Calcium sources include dairy products and vegetables, or supplements. Calcium supplements should be taken in divided doses, such as 600 mg twice per day. I suggest that my patients take calcium citrate such as Citracal® or Caltrate® for better absorption and fewer gastrointestinal side effects. Vitamin D can be obtained in the diet from fortified milk and cereals or saltwater fish. Given that the average American obtains a fraction of the necessary vitamin D from foods or the sun, it is recommended that all women take at least 800 international units or IU of vitamin D in the form of cholecalciferol daily. Vitamin D can be taken in very large doses with no side effects.

What are the pharmacological treatments for osteoporosis?

Alendronate and Risedronate

Both alendronate (Fosamax®) and risedronate (Actonel®) increase bone density and decrease bone loss associated with osteoporosis. Studies of menopausal women report a substantial decrease in the risk for fractures in the spine and hip.

Alendronate and risedronate must be taken on an empty stomach (no food or drink for thirty minutes before or after). In addition, patients should not lie down for half an hour after taking the drug. Bisphosphonates may cause gastrointestinal disturbance, such as nausea and acid reflux. Pain in the stomach and in muscles has also been reported.

Ibandronate

Ibandronate (Boniva®) can be taken as a once-a-month oral dose or once every three months by intravenous injection. Both routes have been associated with significant decreases in both hip and vertebral fractures. Boniva® should also be taken on an empty stomach with the patient sitting or standing for one hour after ingestion. By contrast, intravenous Boniva® is given in the physician's office over two minutes. It avoids the problem with acid reflux or diseases that preclude absorption of the oral form.

Raloxifine

Raloxifine (Evista®), a selective estrogen receptor modulator (SERM), produces some of the same benefits as ERT, without the side effects. Raloxifine is used both to prevent and to treat osteoporosis. Studies show it prevents bone loss and reduces the risk for spinal fractures. In addition to small increases in bone mass in sites typically associated with osteoporosis, raloxifine improves bone density throughout the body.

Raloxifine is given in daily doses of sixty milligrams. Possible side effects include blood clots, hot flashes, and leg cramps.

Calcitonin-salmon

Calcitonin-salmon (Miacalcin®) is a synthetic compound that is chemically identical to the calcitonin found in salmon. Human calcitonin is a hormone secreted by the thyroid gland that helps regulate calcium and bone remodeling. Calcitonin-salmon has been shown to slow bone loss, increase spinal bone mass, and reduce the risk for spinal fractures in menopausal women.

Because calcitonin cannot be properly digested, it is given as an injection or nasal spray. Injectable calcitonin-salmon can be dosed 50 to 100 IU daily. Dosage of the nasal spray is 200 IU daily. The nasal spray may cause a runny nose, nasal soreness, itching, dryness, and crusts.

Synthetic parathyroid hormone

Injectable synthetic parathyroid hormone (Forteo®) is used to treat postmenopausal women at high risk for fracture. A twenty-nine microgram dose is self-injected into the thigh or abdomen directly under the skin once daily with a dial pen for up to twenty-four months. This drug acts on bone-building cells (osteoblasts) to stimulate new bone growth and increase bone mineral density.

Zoledronic acid

In August 2007, the Food and Drug Administration (FDA) approved zoledronic acid (Reclast®) for the treatment of osteoporosis in postmenopausal women. This medication is given intravenously once a year. It must be given in either an office setting or hospital equipped for intravenous drips. Patients must be well hydrated before receiving Reclast®. In rare cases, women receiving this treatment have experienced deterioration (osteonecrosis) of the jaw. Prior to treatment, an oral examination should be performed. **Side effects** include fever, muscle pain, flu like symptoms, and headache.

It always amazes me when one of my eighty-year-old patients refuses to undergo a bone density study on the grounds that she plays tennis, swims, and goes dancing twice a week. She then breaks a hip by tripping on the stairs in her house, and ends up spending the remainder of her life in a nursing home. In contrast, I have patients who constantly complain of arthritic back, hip, and knee pain, whose bone density studies are perfectly normal.

Finally, do not forget that your spouse or boyfriend can develop osteoporosis as well, and men are rarely tested for the disease. You do not know what your fracture risk is unless you undergo a bone density study, so call your doctor's office and schedule one today.

For more information about osteoporosis, visit the National Osteoporosis Foundation at *www.nof.org.*

Chapter 14

Be Informed: The Surgical Consultation

A forty-four-year-old woman presents at my office with a six-month history of bleeding and spotting for two out of every four weeks of each month. She is diagnosed with a uterine polyp by pelvic ultrasound. She then returns for a preoperative consultation prior to her scheduled hysteroscopy, dilatation and curettage. I am about to obtain an **informed consent** from the patient, but before I am able to do this, I need to discuss the following items.

Many women who come in for their preoperative consultations have never had surgery in the past. That is why it is very important that your physician explain exactly what procedure is to be performed. If it is a simple outpatient procedure such as a hysteroscopy (viewing the inside of the uterus) or a cone biopsy of the cervix (removing part of the cervix because of dysplasia), have the physician show you exactly what is going to be done with the use of diagrams and/or models. If the surgery is a hysterectomy, make sure that you understand exactly what is going to be removed and what is going to remain during the surgery. For instance, most patients are under the false assumption that a hysterectomy always involves the removal of the ovaries and cervix, and that they are going to go through menopause. When I perform hysterectomies, I usually leave part of the cervix in place, in order to prevent pelvic prolapse in later years. Similarly, unless a patient is very close to menopause or has already entered menopause, I will usually leave the ovaries in. This prevents surgical menopause and all of its untoward symptoms.

After discussing the actual procedure itself, you must discuss the alternatives to surgery with your doctor. For instance, say that you are experiencing heavy bleeding that is now lasting seven to ten days each month, and your ultrasound shows only small fibroids. Before jumping on the surgical bandwagon, have your physician explain alternative treatments for prolonged bleeding, such as birth control pills or a progestin for a few days out of each month. Your doctor may also place a Mirena® intrauterine device inside your uterus, a simple office procedure, which will significantly decrease your bleeding. By discussing medical therapy for controlling the bleeding problem, you may not only save yourself time away from work and your loved ones, but you will also save money.

After discussing alternatives, the risks versus the benefits of the procedure must be discussed. The risk of any major gynecologic surgery includes but is not limited to damage to the bladder, bowel, ureters, rectum, and major blood vessels. All of these consequences may occur during open surgery (in which the abdomen is cut), laparoscopic surgery, and vaginal surgery. If the bladder is damaged during a hysterectomy because of scar tissue from three previous cesarean sections, you may need to go home with a catheter in your bladder and a bag attached to your leg for ten days. The catheter will then be removed in your doctor's office. You will then need to undergo a retrograde cystogram, in which the bladder is filled with dye and X-rays are taken to ensure that the bladder tear has healed.

Because the bowel, both large and small, surrounds the female pelvic organs, I find that it is imperative that all my patients undergoing either laparoscopy or open laparotomy to remove one or more organs undergo bowel preparation one day prior to their surgery. For my patients, this involves drinking an entire twelve-ounce bottle of magnesium citrate, followed by a clear diet after lunch on the day prior to surgery. This ensures that the bowel is completely cleaned out and collapsed. Consequently, if the bowel is injured during the surgery, it can be repaired easily on the spot, without worrying about stool spilling into the abdomen and causing a massive infection known as peritonitis. I also advise my patients who are undergoing any major abdominal surgery to shave their pubic area and wash the entire abdomen with Hibiclens®, an over-the-counter antibacterial wash, the day before surgery in order to prevent skin infections.

Two major complications of any surgery include bleeding and infection. Bleeding can occur in bloody procedures such as myomectomies, in which the uterus is cut open in multiple locations to remove fibroids and then resutured. In order to avoid such large losses of blood, I sometimes employ a cell-saver machine, in which the lost blood is suctioned into a machine that washes it and returns it to the patient. It is like an autotransfusion. Make sure that you stop all aspirin, ibuprofen, and vitamin E two weeks prior to the surgery. Coumadin, Plavix®, and other blood thinners should also be stopped for at least two weeks. Infection is avoided by using preoperative antibiotics. Make sure that you let your physician know if you have a condition such as mitral valve prolapse, a heart valve, or a hip replacement, which will require prophylactic antibiotics. In order to promote proper healing of wounds, and to prevent wound infections, it is imperative that smokers **stop smoking** at least a month prior to surgery until six weeks after surgery.

Lastly, it is important to know the benefits that your insurance covers when it comes to surgical procedures. In our trying economy, it is imperative that you know what your insurance deductible and/or copay will be for your doctor, the hospital or outpatient center, and the surgical assistant. You do not want to be stuck paying bills two to three months after your procedure. Also, many insurance companies will charge less of copay or no copay at all if your procedure is done in a freestanding outpatient center or physician's office. If the procedure is being performed in your doctor's office and the doctor will be using drugs for sedation or anesthesia, make sure that the office has been accredited by the state medical board to perform surgery and that the office is stocked with equipment and medication in case of a medical emergency.

Now that you are prepared with all of the appropriate questions, you can enter your surgical consultation with confidence.

Chapter 15

Pancreatic Cancer: A Silent Epidemic

I could not think of a better way to end this book than with a chapter dedicated to my mother, Sharyn, who died after a courageous two-year battle with pancreatic cancer in October 2007. Before my mother's unexpected diagnosis, I knew very little about the disease that takes the lives of thousands of people each year. My mother was one of the lucky ones. I had diagnosed her cancer in my office as a complete mistake. She was relatively asymptomatic, except for constipation. When my ultrasonographer placed the probe on her upper abdomen, a four centimeter mass in the head of her pancreas lit up on the screen. She was able to undergo chemotherapy and radiation therapy before the cancer had metastasized.

Most pancreatic cancer patients typically die of the disease within three months of diagnosis. Only **4 percent** of pancreatic cancer patients are alive in five years. We rarely hear about pancreatic cancer unless celebrities such as Michael Landon, Luciano Pavarotti, and Patrick Swayze have been stricken with this disease. Randy Pausch, a computer science professor from Carnegie Mellon University, made headlines with his "Last Lecture" on YouTube. Through perseverance, he has created worldwide awareness of the disease, including its lack of research funding by the federal government and minimal improvement in life expectancy over the last two decades.

Pancreatic cancer is the fourth-leading cause of cancer death overall, according to the American Cancer Society. Nearly 38,000 Americans will be diagnosed with cancer of the pancreas during 2008, and 34,000 will die from the disease.

The pancreas is an organ in the upper abdomen, located beneath the stomach and adjacent to the first portion of the small intestine, known as the duodenum. The pancreas is composed of glands that are responsible for a wide variety of tasks. The glandular functions of the pancreas can be divided into the following two categories: the exocrine glands, which secrete enzymes that help in the digestion of food as it moves through the intestines; and the endocrine glands, which secrete hormones such as insulin. Insulin assists in the process of using sugar as an energy source and controls levels of sugar in the bloodstream.

The pancreas can be divided into the following four anatomical sections:

1. Head – The rightmost portion that lies adjacent to the duodenum (beginning of the small intestine)
2. Uncinate process – An extension of the head of the pancreas
3. Body – The middle portion of the pancreas
4. Tail – The leftmost portion of the pancreas that lies adjacent to the spleen

What are the risk factors for pancreatic cancer?

1. Cigarette smoking
2. Advanced age
3. Chronic pancreatitis, usually from excessive alcohol intake
4. Diabetes
5. Family history of pancreatic cancer

How is pancreatic cancer diagnosed?

The main symptoms of pancreatic cancer include the following: pain in the abdomen, upper back, or both; nausea; weight loss; loss of appetite; abdominal swelling; diarrhea; fatty bowel movements that float in water; new-onset diabetes; and jaundice (yellow skin and eyes). Because the symptoms of pancreatic cancer are often confused with other gastrointestinal disorders such as pancreatitis, cholecystitis (gallbladder disease), or hepatitis (inflammation of the liver) to name a few, it is usually discovered at an advanced stage.

Many of my patients present with family histories of a parent or close relative who succumbed to the disease. I perform a CEA and CA 19-9 blood antigen test on them yearly, along with an ultrasound of the pancreas, gallbladder, and liver. This ultrasound should be performed on a patient who has been fasting for at least six hours. In this way, I can pick up a cancer of the pancreas before any symptoms arise. Many insurance companies will not cover the above testing because they consider it "experimental." Regardless of the price, these tests, which amount to a few hundred dollars, can save your life.

If patients are lucky enough to have their cancer diagnosed before it has metastasized, they may be candidates for a Whipple procedure.

A Whipple procedure (pancreatoduodenectomy) is still the most common procedure for surgically treating pancreatic cancer. This is a radical surgical procedure, often lasting five to eight hours in experienced hands, which involves removing the malignant part of the pancreas and rerouting the stomach and the bile ducts from the liver to the small intestine. Recovery time for this procedure is several weeks, and there can be multiple complications.

Medical treatment

There are no standard recommendations for chemotherapy, but there are a multitude of clinical trials in which one can enroll. For locally advanced pancreatic cancer that cannot be surgically removed safely, a combination of chemotherapy and radiation therapy or chemotherapy alone may be offered. This treatment remains controversial, and various centers have different recommendations based on a number of factors, such as size of the tumor, metastases, and symptoms.

Chemotherapy is the cornerstone of treatment of pancreatic cancer that is locally advanced or metastatic. The chemotherapy agent most commonly used in this setting is gemcitabine, which is often combined with taxotere and Xelota®. This combination is known as GTX. Patients often respond to this treatment for up to twelve months, as seen by tumor regression on CAT scans and PET scans. Most of the time, the tumor becomes resistant, and once again begins to grow.

Gemcitabine (Gemzar®) is given intravenously once a week for seven weeks (or until toxicity limits treatment), and then the patient is given one week off. Cycles are then resumed of gemcitabine once a week for three weeks in a row, followed by one week off. This drug has direct effects on the cancer cells, and is usually given alone for the treatment of metastatic pancreatic cancer. Side effects include fatigue, anemia, and nausea.

Fluorouracil (5 –FU) is usually given intravenously as a continuous infusion, using a medication pump. This drug has direct effects on the cancer cells, and is usually used in combination with radiation therapy because it makes cancer cells more sensitive to the effects of radiation. The side effects include fatigue, diarrhea, mouth sores, and hand-and-foot syndrome (redness, peeling, and pain on the palms of the hands and the soles of the feet).

Xeloda® or capecitabine is given orally and is converted by the body to a compound similar to 5-FU. Capecitabine has similar effects on the cancer cells as 5-FU, and is also generally used in combination with radiation therapy. Side effects are similar to intravenous continuous infusion of 5-FU.

Radiation therapy

Radiation therapy is treatment that uses high-energy X-rays targeted at the cancer to kill cancer cells or to keep them from growing. For pancreatic cancer cases, radiation therapy is usually given in conjunction with chemotherapy.

The goals of radiation therapy are as follows:

1. Shrink the tumor prior to surgery to make it easier to resect.
2. Kill cancer cells that cannot be surgically removed to reduce the risk of the cancer returning or spreading.
3. Treat tumors that cannot be surgically removed and that are causing symptoms such as pain or jaundice.

Typically, radiation treatments are given five days a week, for up to six weeks. Each treatment lasts only a few minutes and is completely painless. However, some patients may experience abdominal discomfort during the last few weeks of therapy or for several months following completion of treatment.

The main side effects of radiation therapy include mild skin irritation, loss of appetite, nausea, diarrhea, or fatigue. These side effects may persist for months, particularly nausea, indigestion, and diarrhea.

Pancreatic cancer is a devastating disease, which attacks with very few warning signs. Increased research funding is paramount to both prevent and treat this disease. If you are interested in learning more about pancreatic cancer, please go to *www.pancan.org* or *www. lustgarten.org.*

Glossary of Commonly Used Terms

atrophic: thin.

atypia: abnormally appearing cells.

biopsy: a sample of tissue.

breakthrough bleeding: uterine bleeding secondary to the abrupt withdrawal of either estrogen or progesterone.

CIN: cervical intraepithelial neoplasia—a precancerous condition of the cervix caused by human papillomavirus.

colposcopy: examination of the cervix and vagina with a specialized microscope.

cone biopsy: a surgical procedure to treat cervical dysplasia, in which a cone-shaped portion of the cervix is cut.

contraception: birth control method.

curettage: the process of scraping either the cervix or uterus to obtain a tissue sample.

cyst: sac-like structure filled with fluid or solid debris.

cystocele: protrusion of the bladder into the vagina.

detrusor muscle: main muscle of the bladder.

dysplasia: abnormal tissue development, which may be precancerous.

ectopic pregnancy: pregnancy occurring outside of the uterus.

endometriosis: the presence of endometrial tissue in locations outside of the uterus.

endometrium: the inside lining of the uterus, which sheds during menstruation.

fibroid: smooth muscle tumor of the uterus, usually benign.

hyperplasia: overgrowth of tissue.

hysterectomy: surgical removal of the uterus and cervix.

hysteroscopy: looking into the uterine cavity with a hollow tube lighted instrument.

incontinence: the involuntary loss of urine.

intrauterine device (IUD): A T-shaped device that may contain progesterone or copper. It remains in the uterus for a number of years.

Kegel's exercises: contraction of the pelvic muscles to prevent laxity of the supporting structures of the bladder, uterus, rectum, and vagina. These exercises are performed by tightening the muscles surrounding the vagina.

laparoscopy: a minimally invasive operative technique that uses small tubular instruments and small abdominal incisions to look and operate inside of the abdomen. This procedure is performed under general anesthesia.

laparotomy: an invasive operation requiring an abdominal incision.

LAVH: laparoscopic-assisted vaginal hysterectomy. The uterus is removed through the vagina.

LEEP: loop electrosurgical excision procedure. Removes a cone-shaped area of the cervix to treat and cure cervical dysplasia.

mittelschmerz: pain associated with ovulation.

myoma: same as fibroid. Benign muscle tumor of the uterus.

myomectomy: removal of uterine fibroids.

neoplasia: scientific term for a group of diseases commonly called tumor or cancer.

oophorectomy: removal of an ovary.

Pap smear: sample of the cervix and vagina used as a screening test for cervical cancer.

prolapse: protrusion of the bladder, rectum, or uterus into the vagina secondary to loss of pelvic floor supports.

rectocele: protrusion of the rectum into the vagina.

salpingectomy: the removal of a fallopian tube.

salpingoophorectomy: removal of an ovary and fallopian tube.

stress urinary incontinence (SUI): the involuntary loss of urine secondary to increased abdominal pressure that occurs with laughing, straining, and jumping.

supracervical hysterectomy: surgical removal of the uterus without the cervix.

tubal ligation: tying the fallopian tubes as a method of contraception.

urethral sling: device placed surgically under the urethra to prevent stress urinary incontinence.

urge incontinence: the involuntary loss of urine due to uncontrollable contractions of the bladder muscle.

uterine prolapse: protrusion of the uterus into the vagina.

vaginal hysterectomy: removal of the uterus and cervix through the vagina without an abdominal incision.

References

http://womenshealth.about.com/cs/annualgynexam/

www.womenshealth.gov/faq/birthcont.htm

www.medicinenet.com/birth-control/article.htm

www.go2planb.com/ForConsumers/Index/aspx

www.mayoclinic.com/health/morning-after-pill/AN00592

www.gardasil.com

www.cdc.gov/std/HPV/STDFact-HPV.htm

www.Herpes.com

www.cdc.gov/Std/Herpes/STDFact-Herpes.htm

www.medicinenet.com/yeast_vaginitis/article.htm

www.4women.gov/faq/yeastinfect.htm

www.ovarian-cysts.com

www.4women.gov.faq/ovarian_cysts.htm#2

www.breastcancer.org

www.cancer.gov/cancerinfo/types/breast

http://womenshealth.about.com/od/hysterectomy/Hysterectomy and Alternatives.htm

www.fda.gov.fdac/features/2001/601_tech.html

www.urinary-incontinence.org

www.mayoclinic.com/health/urinary-incontinence/DS00404

www.womentowomen.com/menopause/postmenopausalbleeding.aspx

www.medicinenet.com/script/main/art.asp?articlekey=51868

www.hormone-replacement-therapy.net/about.htm

www.womentowomen.com/bioidentical-hrt/bioidenticalhormones.aspx

www.nlm.nih.gov/medlineplus/osteoporosis.html

www.nof.org

www.surgeryencylopedia.com/Pa-St/Presurgical-Testing.html

www.healthline.com/galecontent/presurgical-testing

www.pancreaticcancer.org

www.cancer.gov/cancerinfo/wyntk/pancreas